7 Questions You Must Ask When Hospitalized

From a Nurse Who's Been There & Done That!

Debra Lee James, BSN,RN,HNB-BC

DEDICATION

This is written in memory of my grandmother, Arvalean Elizabeth-Marya Lee. À Beautiful Soul lost to Alzheimer-related complications. Im sorry I wasn't as assertive then, as I am now... perhaps your Transition would have been more serene.

This is written in honor of all patients and their families. May you be encouraged to fully advocate for your Loved Ones and yourselves. Let the days of "because I'm the professional and I know best" be forever banished to "Never, NeverLet-It-Be-Said Land."

CONTENTS

ACKNOWLEDGMENTS

To my fellow Angels in human disguise, don't stop fighting for your patients. Demand #SafeStaffingRatios because #SafeStaffingSavesLives. To my #NursesTakeDC crew: keep working to #SavePat!!

To My Family of Origin and My Family of Choice, thank-you for the love, support, advice, encouragement, food, money, late-night phone calls, adversity, funny text messages, reality checks, and even the stinkeyes. I have learned valuable lessons in all situations.

To "Muad'Dib", thank-you those many years ago for sharing your personal family story with me before ever mentioning it to the public. That one phone call is a pivotal vector in my journey.

To My Wonder-Full, Loving, Long-Suffering Husband. Thank-you for loving me through my best/worst/sleep-deprived/demanding/disconnected/perfectionist selves. I love you so much for making me laugh and loving me off of the edge.

INTRODUCTION - MY "WHY"

Hello, my name is Debra Lee James and I'm a nurse. I've worked at the bedside for 10+ years working with a variety of patients, from Telemetry to Med-Surg, Sundowners to Alzheimer's, "new lease on life" to "actively dying." There are some things I've learned over the years. (1) When family is called in after a patient dies, the first question asked 98% of the time: 'Did my loved one die alone? Was someone there with them at the end?' (2) Never assume the status of the **other person** permanently parked in the patient's room. (3) Family involvement affects patient outcomes ... for good or bad.

I've also learned that **many** patients do not ask questions about their care for a variety of reasons. Elders, typically, don't want to appear to be challenging the physician which is considered disrespectful. Women either don't want to seem bossy, or perhaps ignorant of "the obvious." Men don't want to appear ignorant or weak. There are also cultural issues that can lead to misunderstanding, misinformation, and mistrust.

As a patient, I've learned that being a nurse does not always lead to professional courtesy ... usually quite the opposite. Often nurses caring for me view me as a potential threat **because** I'm asking questions. I am in no way questioning their knowledge or integrity. I just want answers regarding information that I would regularly provide to my patients. Besides, as nurses we're supposed to provide patients with knowledge for empowerment and informed decision-making.

Having been on both sides of the hospital bed with experiences bad and good, I've learned seven crucial questions that need to be asked and answered, in order for the best possible outcomes to occur. Here they are:

1. Why am I being admitted?

2. What admission status am I receiving?

3. Who are my care team members?

4. What test, scan, procedure, etc. is being ordered and why?

5. What is my plan of care?

6. Are generic medications being substituted for my brand name medications?

7. What are ALL of my options?

These questions are in no particular order, because every situation is different and has different priorities. Let's explore each of these questions together, shall we?

"Come along and ride on a fantastic voyage!"

~ *Fantastic Voyage*, by Lakeside © Sony/ATV Music Publishing LLC, Warner/Chappell Music, Inc.

Question 1 - Why Am I Being Admitted?

This question may seem like a blinding flash of the obvious. However, you'd be surprised how many patients and/or families cannot answer this question. As the nurse, I already know the answer from the report I received prior to admission or prior to starting my shift. I still ask the question. On occasions too numerous to count, the answer to that question is essentially a narration of the events leading up to the Emergency visit, concluding with some version of *'and so the doctor said I'm being admitted.'*

Now you may be thinking to yourself, of course the Emergency doctor tells the patient why they're being admitted. Well consider this, on a "good" day any Emergency department has visits involving everything from a splinter to an unexpected birth to a gun shot wound (GSW). During evaluation, there is not always a preferential placement for the lesser traumas, meaning they can be on a gurney next to a serious trauma with only a thin curtain between. I know form first-hand experience that one can be easily distracted by another's situation to the point of not quite paying full attention to the information being provided by the doctor. I also know that patients who feel they are being "blown off" by staff generally tune out after a time.

Most recently that experience played out in the Emergency department at Bellevue Hospital in NYC, where I discovered that at shift change all non-patients are removed from/prevented entry to the department. My bad luck to fall down the up escalator at Penn Station just prior to shift change. Aside from the fact that my Intern pretty much ignored my statements and questions causing me to say whatever got me discharged, I became concerned about the woman next to me. She spoke almost no English and her grandson(?) who interpreted for her was escorted out at shift change. Come to think of it, I don't remember him or anyone else being allowed back in after shift change. My Spanish isn't great but I knew enough to learn she was very hungry after spending the day without any food. I finally got someone to verify that she could eat, and gave her half of my sandwich (which I had no interest in finishing) and my can of soda provided by the department.

Anyone who can go through a similar ordeal and still retain everything told to them during that time until they are admitted, I tip my hat to you. You are an extraordinary person with the presence of Buddha and the self-control of a Vulcan. For the rest of us, it's fairly easy to see the possible reasons for not knowing exactly why we are being admitted.

Why do you need this specific information? Because your admitting diagnosis drives your plan of care, your treatments, even your meals. Let's say your admitting diagnosis is heart failure flare up (aka CHF exacerbation.) You may be placed on a fluid restriction, meaning that habit of sipping soda from dinner to bedtime is going to be sorely missed. Also, knowing this information helps you better understand if the plan of care is helpful, harmful, or non-existent. You know what is expected of you and what is expected from your care providers.

FYI if you are told that surgery is on the horizon, find out what practitioners are to be involved and **make sure your insurance is accepted by each practitioner.** We had a situation where the clinic had changed anesthesia practices. Imagine our surprise (and we were not alone) when we were told anesthesia was not covered by insurance. Say WHAAAAAAAT??? The anesthesia practice was in the process of accepting other insurances, but either they didn't realize how long the process would take, or no one bothered to check beforehand what main insurances are used in the area. Either way, not a happy first encounter. You've had enough surprises up to this point. You don't need a surprise bill showing up in your mailbox.

Question 2 - What Admission Status Am I Receiving?

Again, another seemingly blinding flash of the obvious, yes? Not so fast - about 5-6 years ago, hospitals came up with an interesting admission status called **"Observation."** Most hospitals charge a flat fee each day of admission that lasts beyond midnight. I have had patients given discharge orders at 3 am; some were ready and eager to leave, others were sent on their way to free up a bed for waiting admissions. Thus became the hybrid (my word) admission status of "Observation."

"Observation" essentially means you are placed in a hospital bed, but you're still considered to be an **outpatient**. Why does this matter? It's all about fees. Rather than pay a daily flat rate fee, you can be charged **BY THE HOUR.** No need for a vision check, you did in fact, just read **BY THE HOUR**. That means your room is assigned a special hourly rate, and medications, meals, treatments, etc. are charged individually on a per use basis. I believe you can agree with me when I say this is a creative way for hospitals to manifest more income. Not making accusations, just expressing my opinion.

I've had patients with this admission status who were self-pay and asked to be released in the wee hours, rather than waiting for the doctor to arrive mid-morning simply to sign the discharge paperwork. Legally, they are leaving AMA (against medical advice.) Morally, should they be charged with additional fees when they don't have insurance and are footing the bill themselves? This is just one ethical dilemma that nurses struggle to deal with every shift. How does a nurse grapple with this scenario while handling a patient with dementia, a patient with a very fast irregular heart beat, a patient fresh from surgery, a patient on end-of-life care, and a patient that insists hospital and Hilton are one and the same. Another reason to push Congress for mandated safe staffing of nurse-to-patient ratios.

FYI if you are told that surgery, or a special procedure is on the horizon, find out what practitioners are to be involved and **make sure your insurance is accepted by each practitioner.** We had a situation where the clinic had changed anesthesia practices. Imagine our surprise (and we were not alone) when we were told anesthesia was not covered by insurance. Say WHAAAAAAAT??? The anesthesia practice was in the process of accepting other insurances, but either they didn't realize how long the process would take, or no one bothered to check beforehand the main insurances used in the area. Either way, not a happy first encounter. You've had enough surprises up to this point. You don't need a surprise bill showing up in your mailbox.

QUESTION 3 - WHO ARE MY CARE TEAM MEMBERS?

Your care team consists of the people and/or departments that provide clinical services during your hospital stay. This team's function is to coordinate care across the various departments and disciplines to provide your best possible outcome, with little or no repetition. It's fair to say the 'basic' care team includes (1) the treating doctor(s), (2) the Charge or Resources nurse for the unit, (3) the primary nurse responsible for your care during the shift, and (4) the nurse's assistant, aide or technician.

Typically your hospital room will have some sort of status board with your name, your diagnosis, any safety concerns (e.g. high fall risk, hearing-impaired, etc.) your doctor's name, the names of your primary nurse and aide/technician. The information that may change each shift is expected to be updated by the on-coming team members. Every team member is expected to introduce themselves at the beginning of each shift, as well as talk up the oncoming shift at the end of their shift.

On a perfect day this works extremely well.

However, as in the rest of life, perfection is rarely a daily event. There are times when, for whatever reason, wrong or incomplete information is passed from one shift to the next. Case in point: I had been given report on my module (aka patient group) one night, only to find out after the previous shift nurse had gone home, that one of my patient's had a positive TB skin test, had not had the results explained to her, and had not been moved into a specific type of isolation room for definite or suspected TB infection. Family members were going in and out of the room without isolation gowns or masks, and the patient was in tears thinking she would soon die, and may have even infected an infant grandchild that had visited. It took some time, several hours actually, to calm down the patient by explaining in detail what the skin test results actually represent, reassuring the family, and moving the patient to the proper isolation room. Hmmmm looks like that 8pm medication pass (med pass) is going to be late.

Did the previous shift nurse intentionally not tell me about the test results? Did that nurse believe she had given me the information? Did another nurse receive the information and forget to tell the patient's nurse because it wasn't their patient? Who knows? It happened and can't be undone. There are also times when the oncoming nurse is told about a prescription written by a doctor for a patient. When it's time for the next med pass, that new med isn't showing up on the patient's list. OK, maybe the pharmacy hasn't had time to fill the order or send the med to the unit.

Another hour passes, so a call is made to pharmacy at which point you are told there are no new orders. You check the patient chart, praying for the miracle that the order is there but was never sent to pharmacy. There is no order. You review all orders hoping that what you're looking for is buried amongst the many hand-written orders. No ... it's not there. Did the doctor forget? Was there a technical glitch with the computer systems? Was the order placed in the wrong chart? None of that matters, because now you have to start making phone calls to fix the situation in a (hopefully) timely manner.

Bottom line: you need to know the name and designation of each member of your care team. Doctor's have business cards on them 90% of their waking lives. Ask for one. It will provide you with their name, specialty and contact information for future reference. For convenience, keep an empty letter size envelope next to your bed to hold all business cards. You can make notes on the envelope or directly on the cards as memory refreshers.

When anyone comes in your room to provide care, ask them their name & job. Ask them, nicely, to update the status board if needed. Then **formally introduce yourself to that team member.** Why? You want to be recognized and respected **as a real, living, breathing person** and <u>NOT</u> an assignment, a room number, an illness, a challenge, or a distraction. You want to be recognized as an individual. It's difficult for most people to meet someone on such a vulnerable level (being a patient) and not have a vested interest in their well-being once they acknowledge the person of **you.** And you definitely want that acknowledgment to work for your benefit.

QUESTION 4 - WHAT TEST, SCAN, PROCEDURE, ETC. IS BEING ORDERED AND WHY?

During a typical hospital stay it's normal to have your blood drawn and tested each morning, especially if you're taking blood thinners, to make sure the medicine is working. It's normal to have your blood tested at specific times when being treated for a serious infection, again to make sure the medicine is working. X-rays for bone or fall injuries, CT for possible stroke, ECG for heart problems, each perfectly normal and expected, right? At what point does the testing become excessive or unnecessary?

At one time my grandmother, Arvalean, was found at home, initially unconscious and was taken by ambulance to the hospital. She was mildly confused, very weak and after some testing was diagnosed with dehydration and a bladder infection. Made sense to me and I learned that confusion can be caused by a bladder infection. One thing kept bugging me - why did my grandmother need a spinal tap in the E.R. and why couldn't I stay with her when it was performed? Over the next several days blood work, x-rays, CT scans, MRI's and physical exams continued.

Still, no one in the family knew all the doctors involved in her care or who was ordering what tests and why. The camel-back-breaking straw happened when one of the doctors insisted on performing another spinal tap. Are you kidding me? Needless to say, after a "family meeting" at the hospital where no concrete reason was given for the second spinal tap, that test was cancelled.

A case of miscommunication between doctors? A case of CYA in the hopes of avoiding a lawsuit? A case of "her insurance is awesome so let's milk this for as long as possible"? We'll never know, but I often wonder the consequences of all those additional, but perhaps unnecessary, tests and scans.

When you know all the members of the care team it's much easier to track the orders. And while you sign a general consent to treat form on admission, some procedures require further consent (e.g. transfusion, CT scan, invasive procedures, etc.) Some tests involve injecting dye that may affect your regular medication use; is it worth it? Some tests bombard your body with huge doses of electromagnetic energy or radiation. Some healthcare professionals say with each test your cells become more susceptible to genetic changes. Is it worth it?

Bear in mind that all those specialized tests may not be covered by insurance, or may have a limit in the number of tests performed each year. When a test is suggested, ask ***WHY**, ***WHAT** are the consequences of having and not having, *__WHO__ is performing the test and what are their qualifications, *__WHEN__ does the test need to be done? Can the test be performed as an outpatient, which is often less expensive? Remember, you do have the right to refuse treatment as long as you're willing to accept the consequences of not being treated. <u>Be an informed decision-maker</u>.

QUESTION 5 - WHAT IS MY PLAN OF CARE?

Now that you know all the players and their roles, how does it all come together? This is where the care plan comes into play. This is where the nuts and bolts of your care are spelled out for the entire care team. Contrary to popular belief, this game plan is meant to be dynamic, not static, to adjust to the patient's changing health status over the length of the hospital stay. First and foremost your care plan, if properly prepared, has your primary admitting diagnosis. I say primary, because most patients tend to have more than one health issue especially elder patients. The primary diagnosis is the reason for admission and drives the focus of treatment. Unfortunately, there are times when there is no inkling of a primary diagnosis. What there is, is a listing of each and every health issue with which the patient has ever been diagnosed.

Let me walk you through this. Patient "A" has an admitting diagnosis of <u>Heart Failure Exacerbation (flare-up)</u>. The nurse's plan of care will include a daily weight (to monitor for water retention), measuring of intake & output (to monitor fluid balance), possibly a fluid intake restriction and other **measurable** activities to correct the flare-up such that patient "A" will be back to their usual activities as soon as possible. Patient "B", on the other hand, has this admitting diagnosis: <u>diabetes</u>, <u>macular degeneration</u>, <u>acid reflux</u> <u>and</u> <u>the</u> <u>always</u> <u>popular</u> <u>ambulatory dysfunction</u>. What, you may ask is ambulatory dysfunction? It's a fancy way of saying the patient has problems walking. How does the nurse determine the plan of care with measurable goals? The diabetes is chronic and unless there are wild swings in blood sugar levels, what and how do you measure improvement? Macular degeneration is a chronic illness that does not improve. There's no way to measure the speed at which the patient is losing their vision, and the disease process doesn't exactly move at a known consistent rate. Acid reflux - another chronic condition that when well-managed isn't very measurable. How do you measure stomach acid on a daily basis?

Ambulatory dysfunction. A catch-all term if ever there was one. I've never seen it as an ICD-9 insurance code, but who knows? Maybe it's covered under ICD-10 which is so much more specialized for accuracy. Problems walking is a symptom, not a diagnosis. How can you develop measurable goals when you don't know what's causing the problem(s) with walking? You can't. And yet, care plans will address the issue. **All** care plans will address the issue in terms of something called 'fall risk assessment.' Why? It's one of those lovely little

Medicare reimbursement items that put the fear of The Almighty into hospital administrators and risk assessment professionals as fast as a first-timer's polar bear plunge. Patients are screened for risk of fall typically using a short list of questions with a numerical value assigned to each answer. Once added up, the care plan is adjusted as needed. Of course if the reason for admission is related to a fall, high risk classification is automatic.

So if all the proper procedures are in place and a patient still manages to fall (maybe while in the radiology department, or dialysis center) Medicare reimbursement is not likely to be affected. However, if the proper procedures are **not** in place the hospital can pretty much kiss that reimbursement good-bye. Oh yeah, any injuries that happen due to the fall will also **not** likely be reimbursed by Medicare.

Your care plan **should** also address your spiritual needs. Some facilities place a stronger emphasis on this than other facilities, but faith values can be a critical factor in patient care. I've had patients who are members of Jehovah's Witnesses which meant every care team member had to be aware that the patient would not receive any blood products. I've Muslim, Jewish and Hindu patients who required careful attention to dietary needs. I also had a patient who very reluctantly told me her faith was Paganism. Her reluctance being a result of her E.R. experience that evening with the person doing pre-admission. When she mentioned her faith, she was told by the clerk "That's not a real religion, so I'll put no preference." Are you kidding me??!!! Clerk was completely out of line. Needless to say, much effort on my part was required to regain that patient's trust. Maybe it's easy for me to identify with that patient, because in the area where I live when I say my faith preference is A.M.E. (African Methodist Episcopal) quite often I, too, get the what-tha-heck-is-that??? Look.

The bottom line is the care plan is the blueprint for treatment to improve health and allow discharge as soon as <u>safely</u> possible. You have a right to see the care plan and judge for yourself whether or not it's appropriate and being appropriately used. While you don't need a medical degree or PhD to understand the intricate details of the care plan (although it does make things easier), you do need some basic medical background knowledge. When asking for your copy of your care plan, be respectful, bearing in mind your nurse has more patients than you to care for during their shift. Yes, you have a right to view your care plan, but no, you don't have a right to demand it or threaten staff if you don't get it exactly when you want it. It's that whole fly catching, honey vs. vinegar thing. You remember that saying, right?

QUESTION 6 - ARE GENERIC MEDICATIONS BEING SUBSTITUTED FOR MY BRAND-NAME MEDICATIONS?

"Generics are as effective as brand names, they're just less expensive." True or False? The answer is... YES! Generics are less expensive, but they're becoming less, less expensive. As more and more consumers began opting for generics over brand-names, pharmaceutical companies saw a steady decline in their brand-name profit margins. As such, said companies have increased the cost of generics over the past few years. While the cost of some generics has increased as much as 7,000% consumers remain heavily invested in the generics-are-cheaper mindset. I wonder how long will the cost difference remain significant enough to be acceptable for the average consumer?

Hospitals are heavily invested in stocking generics for a number of reasons. One of the most obvious reasons being cost-savings. I'm not sure of how medications are billed, but I'm fairly certain it varies from one facility to another, and state to state. Riddle me this: if a facility charges the same price whether it's generic or brand-name, is it a)legal and moral, b)legal and immoral, c)illegal and moral, or d)illegal and immoral? That is not to say that this is, or is not hospital protocol. Whatever the case, one generic can substitute for several brand-names, thereby saving costs and saving storage space.

What does this mean for you? If you're like me and have multiple drug and food allergies or issues it could mean the difference between mild stomach problems and anaphylactic reactions that may lead to death. Yes, generics do contain the same primary ingredients as brand-names. The issue is what type of fillers are used. As I walk through a pharmacy, grocery store, or membership store, looking at over the counter (OTC) medications I compare ingredients between generic and brand-name. The main ingredients are essentially the same with maybe slight differences in amounts. So far, so good. However, the filler ingredients (aka other ingredients per manufacturer listing) have some things I can't safely consume.

I'm 100% lactose intolerant (which allegedly got me a write up in a professional journal somewhere because my doctor had never seen a straight line result for lactase enzyme testing.) I have no lactase enzyme in my body and I have no idea when or why it went away. I'm also allergic to high fructose corn syrup, which is used as an inexpensive sweetener in just about everything from fruit juice to electrolyte replacement drinks to cough medicine and chewing gum. Guess what's the number one filler for OTC medications? You guessed it, lactose! These filler ingredients can change at any time. Some generics that I used

to be able to take have had to fall by the wayside
because what once contained zero 'no-no'
ingredients, now after 10 years has been
reformulated to have 'no-no' ingredients.

Kind of like the makers of Sunkist orange soda.
Initially had more caffeine than Mountain Dew, but
caffeine content was not labeled. Consumers found
out, the label included caffeine and a number of
consumers stopped drinking (personally for me it
was the whole bait and switch routine that made me
stop.) The makers decided to go completely
caffeine-free and sales did not exactly skyrocket.
Guess what? Caffeine was added again, with LESS
caffeine content than Mountain Dew AND
appropriately labeled. What do you know? Sales
steadily climbed. Current listing shows 41 mg of
caffeine and 52 **grams** of sugar.

If your provider has written prescriptions with
the annotation "brand name only", that is what you
should be receiving. Remember though, most
facilities have a limited number of brand-name
medications on hand. If your medication is listed
for generic in the hospital formulary you have
three options, 1)contact the prescribing
practitioner and ask if it's safe to take a
generic while hospitalized, 2)take the generic
without contacting your provider, or 3)bring your
brand-name medication with you or have someone
bring it in for you. Any meds brought from home
must be communicated to your care team, especially
your nurse. Full disclosure - I was once
hospitalized post-surgery and none of my
medications were ordered by the surgeon. Rather
than having my husband bring my meds the next day,

I figured a few days without the meds wouldn't be a problem. Due to minor complications my stay was extended by about three days. I soon learned that suddenly stopping Synthroid is a very poor decision that I paid for, for about three weeks. Please be smarter than I was back in the day.

QUESTION 7 - WHAT ARE <u>ALL</u> OF MY OPTIONS?

If information overload causes you to be paralyzed by inaction, be gentle with yourself. Ask about only those issues that are of importance to <u>you</u>. For the rest of us there's no such thing as information overload and we want it **ALL!** There is no way I can make a truly informed decision if information is withheld from me, especially if the withholding is an intentional act. Exactly why is information withheld? There are possibly as many reasons as there are different shoe sizes. Perhaps the care provider realizes the patient will likely not survive some options. Or, maybe the patient's insurance will not cover some options. Or, just maybe, the care provider isn't aware of other options. All believable scenarios.

I offer this story as another possible reason. I had a widowed, elderly patient who was told by a specialist that she had to have a cardiac catheterization (angioplasty, stent placement) that evening or she risked death. I had been told in report that before ANY procedure was to be performed, her son (living in another state) must be contacted. I informed the specialist of same and provided the son's phone number. Meanwhile during my assessment of the patient I was concerned about her anxiety over the procedure. The patient told me she really didn't want to have the procedure. She told me her husband was dead, all of her siblings were dead, and all of her closest friends were dead. Her children were grown, doing well and she didn't really have a good reason for prolonging her life.

I explained that there was no requirement for her to have the procedure. She told me she didn't want to upset her son, or the specialist by going against their wishes. I asked, if you don't have the procedure and die the next day, would you, just before you took your last breath, wish you'd had the procedure? Essentially she said she was ready to die, but she didn't want to go against her son, or anger the specialist by refusing treatment. Now throughout this exchange I'm going back and forth between patient and specialist. On this particular shift said specialist is in **serious** "god-complex" mode. Yelling, throwing things, being verbally abusive to and blaming staff for not having equipment and paperwork ready for this procedure as he had ordered. This situation had me walking a tightrope.

The last time I spoke with the patient I told her that the decision was completely up to her. I assured her that it's her body, she has the final say AND she has the right to refuse treatment as long as she's comfortable with consequences of refusal. She refused and I went skipping down the hall to inform the specialist of her decision. Said specialist was not a happy camper when I made it crystal clear that the patient was absolutely comfortable with risking death.

What does this mean for you? First and foremost, if you are in an emergency situation, **this question does NOT apply to your situation**. An emergency is just that. All bets are off, and you rely on whatever gives you hope that the right people and resources are in the right place at the right time.

When you are told a procedure needs to be performed, the fist question should be, "Is this something that can be done as an outpatient?" As I've stated previously, outpatient procedures tend to be less expensive. The next question should be, "Is there a less invasive procedure that can be done?" Nothing wrong with avoiding any procedure that may have a higher risk for infection. Other questions include:

* Who is performing the procedure and how much experience do they have with this procedure? I remember one time the VA facility I was using expressed excitement over the possibility of removing my gall bladder with new equipment they were just itching to try out. I gracefully declined.

* Is this procedure the industry standard? Again, you don't want to be the proverbial guinea pig.

* What other options exist for this procedure?

* What are the risks of blood loss, further complications, and post-procedure infection with each available option?

* Do I need pre-approval from my insurance for this procedure?

Wow! This is a lot of information and there are likely more specific issues you need to research to address your particular situation. These seven questions are not meant to be used as commandments. These seven questions are not meant to be used to brow-beat, intimidate, or provide the basis for a lawsuit. For that matter, none of the information presented here is meant to take the place of information provided by your doctor, or other qualified healthcare professionals. These seven questions are meant to be used as **a guideline, a resource, and an empowerment tool**. I want each and every person reading this book to feel confident about advocating for yourselves or a Loved One. You **can** do this. I believe in **you**. Stay Blessed!

"Hardships often prepare ordinary people for an extraordinary destiny."
~ C.S. Lewis

ABOUT THE AUTHOR

Debra Lee James is the youngest child born into a military family, and from the beginning has generally danced to the rhythm of her own beat. From challenging and confronting bullies at age four to defiantly obtaining two bachelor's degrees when her Freshman chemistry prof said she was better suited for an associate degree. Whenever someone said "you can't", she generally made them say, "how did you do that?" She earned her first bachelor's degree (BA Sociology, Cum Laude) from Howard University in 1984 where she also received an Air Force commission as a 2nd Lieutenant. She jokes that her mantra is Navy, by birth. Army, by marriage. Air Force, by choice!

She earned her nursing degree (BS Nursing) from The Johns Hopkins University School of Nursing in 2003, and a few months later passed her state licensing exam on the first attempt. She joined the American Holistic Nurses Association in 2004 and passed the certification exam for Holistic Nursing in 2010 also on her first attempt. Debra has practiced holistically for over 10 years at the bedside primarily caring for cardiac/telemetry/med-surg patients. She has also cared for hospice patients, patients in physical rehab, and patients in long-term care facilities.

Debra is the proud owner of Angelic Touch Health & Wellness, LLC, her nurse consulting business. She lives in Maryland with her husband of 22 years and three fur-babies, aka cats.